DOWN'S SYNDROME

SIMPLE REMEDIES FOR DOWN'S SYNDROME

DR. KELSEY LAWSON

Contents

CHAPTER ONE

INTRODUCTION

Down syndrome is a genetic situation in which someone is born with a further copy of chromosome 21. This indicates that they have got a complete of forty seven chromosomes instead of forty six. This may affect how their thoughts and body broaden. Humans diagnosed with Down syndrome have happy and wholesome lives with supportive care.

Down syndrome is a genetic situation wherein people are born with a further chromosome. Most people have 23 pairs of chromosomes inside each mobile in their frame, for an entire of forty six. A person identified with Down syndrome has a further reproduction of chromosome 21, this means that their cells encompass 47 standard chromosomes as opposed to forty six. This modifications the manner their thoughts and body increase.

Down syndrome is a genetic ailment caused even as bizarre mobile department consequences in a similarly full or partial replica of chromosome 21. This extra genetic cloth reasons the developmental adjustments and bodily functions of Down syndrome.

Down syndrome varies in severity amongst people, causing lifelong intellectual incapacity and developmental delays. It's far the maximum common genetic chromosomal illness and cause of studying disabilities in youngsters. It additionally generally causes different scientific abnormalities, together with heart and gastrointestinal troubles.

Higher statistics of Down syndrome and early interventions can greatly growth the exceptional of existence for kids and adults with this illness and help them live beautiful lives.

Down syndrome is a genetic scenario that causes moderate to critical physical and developmental issues.

People with Down syndrome are born with a further chromosome. Chromosomes are bundles of genes, and your body relies on having truely the proper variety of them. With Down syndrome, this greater chromosome results in some of issues that have an effect on you both mentally and physically.

Down syndrome is a lifelong scenario. Despite the fact that it can't be cured, doctors recognize extra about it now than ever. In case your little one has it, getting the right care early on should make a big distinction in assisting them stay a full and sizeable existence.

Down Syndrome signs and symptoms

Down syndrome may additionally have many outcomes, and it's one of a kind for each person. Some will develop as a whole lot as stay almost simply on their private, at the equal time as others will need greater help taking care of themselves.

Intellectual abilities range, however most of the people with Down syndrome have slight to slight troubles with wondering, reasoning, and understanding. They'll examine and choose up new abilties their complete lives, but they may take longer to reap critical desires like taking walks, speakme, and growing social skills.

Human beings with Down syndrome usually generally tend to have wonderful physical competencies in commonplace. The ones may additionally encompass:

Eyes that slant up at the outer corner

Small ears

Flat noses

Protruding tongue

Tiny white spots inside the colored a part of the eyes

Brief neck

Small hands and feet

Brief stature

Free joints

Susceptible muscle tone

Many people with Down syndrome don't have some other fitness troubles, however a few do. Not unusual situations consist of coronary heart problems and hassle listening to and seeing.

Reasons

Human cells commonly contain 23 pairs of chromosomes. One chromosome in each pair comes out of your father, the alternative from your mother.

Down syndrome outcomes even as regular cellular department regarding chromosome 21 occurs. Those cell division abnormalities result in a further partial or complete chromosome 21. This extra genetic material is accountable for the function functions and developmental troubles of Down syndrome. Anyone of three genetic variations can purpose Down syndrome:

Trisomy 21. About 90 5 percent of the time, Down syndrome is because of trisomy 21 — the character has three copies of chromosome 21, as opposed to the same old copies, in all cells. That is due to everyday mobile branch throughout the development of the sperm cell or the egg cellular.

Mosaic Down syndrome. On this unusual form of Down syndrome, a person has only a few cells with a further replica of chromosome 21. This mosaic of everyday and strange cells is as a result of strange cell branch after fertilization.

Translocation Down syndrome. Down syndrome also can arise at the same time as a part of chromosome 21 will become attached (translocated) onto any other chromosome, earlier than or at notion. Those youngsters have the identical vintage two copies of chromosome 21, but similarly they have got extra genetic cloth from chromosome 21 connected to some other chromosome.

There aren't any seemed behavioral or environmental elements that motive Down syndrome.

Is it inherited?

Maximum of the time, Down syndrome isn't inherited. It is because of a mistake in cellular branch throughout early improvement of the fetus.

Translocation Down syndrome can be surpassed from figure to infant. However, only approximately three to four percentage of youngsters with Down syndrome have translocation and only some of them inherited it from really one among their parents.

Even as balanced translocations are inherited, the guardian has some rearranged genetic fabric from chromosome 21 on any other chromosome, but no greater genetic material. This suggests she or he has no signs or signs and symptoms of Down syndrome, but can pass an unbalanced translocation on to children, causing Down syndrome in the youngsters.

Risk factors

Some mother and father have a greater threat of having a infant with Down syndrome. Hazard factors consist of:

Advancing maternal age. A female's possibilities of giving begin to a baby with

Down syndrome increase with age due to the fact older eggs have a extra risk of fallacious chromosome branch. A lady's chance of conceiving a little one with Down syndrome will increase after 35 years of age. However, maximum kids with Down syndrome are born to girls beneath age 35 because more younger ladies have an extended manner more infants.

Being businesses of the genetic translocation for Down syndrome. Both ladies and men can skip the genetic translocation for Down syndrome immediately to their children.

Having had one child with Down syndrome. Mother and father who have one infant with Down syndrome and parents who have a translocation themselves are at an improved hazard of having a few other baby with Down syndrome. A genetic counselor can assist mother and father test the hazard of getting a 2nd baby with Down syndrome.

Headaches

People with Down syndrome may also have a diffusion of complications, some of which turn out to be more distinguished as they grow to be older. Those complications can include:

Coronary heart defects. About half of of the kids with Down syndrome are born with some form of congenital heart infection. The ones coronary coronary heart issues may be lifestyles-threatening and can require surgical treatment in early infancy.

CHAPTER TWO

Gastrointestinal (GI) defects. GI abnormalities arise in some youngsters with Down syndrome and might consist of abnormalities of the intestines, esophagus, trachea and anus. The danger of developing digestive troubles, together with GI blockage, heartburn (gastroesophageal reflux) or celiac ailment, may be prolonged.

Immune problems. Due to abnormalities in their immune structures, people with Down syndrome are at elevated hazard of developing autoimmune issues, a few sorts of cancer, and infectious sicknesses, together with pneumonia.

Sleep apnea. Because of easy tissue and

skeletal modifications that lead to the obstruction of their airlines, youngsters and adults with Down syndrome are at greater hazard of obstructive sleep apnea.

Weight issues. Humans with Down syndrome have a more tendency to be overweight compared with the overall populace.

Spinal problems. Some humans with Down syndrome may additionally have a misalignment of the pinnacle two vertebrae inside the neck (atlantoaxial instability). This circumstance puts them vulnerable to severe damage to the spinal cord from overextension of the neck.

Leukemia. Younger youngsters with Down syndrome have an elevated risk of leukemia.

Dementia. Human beings with Down syndrome have a extensively multiplied hazard of dementia — signs and symptoms and signs and symptoms can also begin round age 50. Having Down syndrome also will growth the threat of growing Alzheimer's disorder.

Extraordinary problems. Down syndrome will also be associated with different fitness situations, along with endocrine problems, dental troubles, seizures, ear infections, and listening to and imaginative and prescient issues.

For human beings with Down syndrome, getting recurring health center treatment and treating troubles at the same time as wanted can help with preserving a healthful way of existence.

Life expectancy

Life spans have elevated dramatically for humans with Down syndrome. Nowadays, someone with Down syndrome can expect to stay greater than 60 years, relying on the severity of health problems.

How is Down syndrome recognized in advance than delivery?

A healthcare enterprise can suspect Down syndrome in the course of being pregnant with prenatal screening tests. They also can diagnose this circumstance sooner or later of being pregnant with diagnostic exams.

Prenatal screening exams

These exams take a look at your danger of having a child with Down syndrome in preference to providing you with a confirmation of a analysis. Screening exams could be a blood take a look at of the birthing determine's blood to search for signs and symptoms of Down syndrome. A few other screening take a look at is an ultrasound. At some point of this imaging check, your issuer will search for symptoms and signs of Down syndrome, like extra fluid inside the returned of your child's neck. It's possible that a screening take a look at may be everyday and no longer display symptoms of Down syndrome whilst the circumstance is gift.

Diagnostic exams during pregnancy

Diagnostic assessments during being pregnant can affirm a Down syndrome analysis. They generally take vicinity after a effective screening take a look at. Diagnostic testing gives greater danger for the birthing figure and the developing fetus. Exams could encompass:

Amniocentesis.

Chorionic villus sampling (CVS).

Percutaneous umbilical blood sampling (PUBS).

Those assessments can hit upon chromosomal modifications that lead to a Down syndrome analysis.

How is Down syndrome recognized after delivery?

After your little one is born, companies look for the physical signs of Down syndrome inside the course of a bodily examination. To affirm the prognosis, your little one's corporation may moreover carry out a blood take a look at referred to as a karyotype take a look at. In this check, your toddler's company will remove a small blood pattern to look at under a microscope. They'll search for an extra twenty first chromosome to diagnose the condition.

What if I find out that the fetus has Down syndrome?

In case you discover the fetus you're carrying has Down syndrome, your groups will direct you to resources that will help you after the begin of your toddler. You could need to participate in counseling or be a part of a help institution. Counselors and assist organizations help you put together for raising a toddler with Down syndrome.

In help companies, you may talk with other dad and mom about their research raising a toddler with Down syndrome. It's a top notch way to percent practical recommendation on managing the scenario, its frustrations and joys. The ones organizations offer a experience of belonging and come up with help, so you comprehend you're not by myself.

There's no remedy for Down syndrome, but treatment is available to assist your infant gain their full ability. Treatment specializes in assisting your little one thrive bodily and mentally. Remedy alternatives need to embody:

Bodily or occupational remedy.

Speech remedy.

Collaborating in special education applications in university.

Treating any underlying scientific conditions.

Carrying glasses for imaginative and prescient troubles or assisted hearing devices for hearing loss.

Prevention

There's no way to save you Down syndrome. In case you're at excessive threat of getting a baby with Down syndrome or you've got already were given one infant with Down syndrome, you can want to are seeking advice from a genetic counselor in advance than turning into pregnant.

A genetic counselor permit you to understand your chances of getting a toddler with Down syndrome. She or he can also explain the prenatal exams which are to be had and assist provide an reason behind the professionals and cons of finding out.

What sources are available for people dwelling with Down syndrome and their households?

There are assets to be had to human beings with Down syndrome and their families. Many families be part of Down syndrome manual organizations to percentage their reviews and methods to help their youngsters stay a healthy, complete lifestyles.

People with Down syndrome will likely need help throughout their lives. Further to ongoing therapies, this may encompass assist with training, employment and dwelling independently. A spread of businesses provide resources to help educate and empower humans residing with Down syndrome and their families.

Conclusion

It may feel overwhelming to look at that your baby has Down syndrome. As you process the news, understand that you're not by myself and that your little one's more chromosome is a part of what makes them specific. You could find manual via your little one's health center treatment team or by using turning into a member of groups for households and caregivers to research extra about the scenario and the way to help your infant grow.

THE END